Break Your Sugar Addiction Recipes

Sugar Free Cooking to
Reset Your Leptin Resistance &
Lose Weight, Get Healthy

Geoff & Vicky Wells

The companion cookbook to
Sugar And The Evil Empire

Copyright© 2015 by Geoff & Vicky Wells

Library of Congress Control Number: 2015905400

All rights reserved

No part of this book may be used or reproduced in any manner whatsoever without prior written permission from the publisher, except for the inclusion of brief quotations in reviews.

Cover Artwork & Design by
Old Geezer Designs

Published in the United States by
Terra Novian Press
an imprint of
DataIsland Software LLC,
Hollywood, Florida

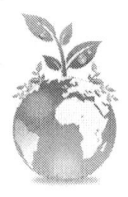

ebooks.geezerguides.com

ISBN 978-0-9772346-1-5

Neither the author nor the publisher assumes responsibility for errors in internet addresses or for changes in the addresses after publication. Nor are they responsible for the content of websites they do not own.

Table of Contents

Foreword 1
Introduction 3

Breakfast 7
Buckwheat Pancakes 8
Multi-Grain Hot Cereal 9
Buckwheat and Almond Flour Blueberry Pancakes 10
Vicky's Sugar-Free Granola 12
Overnight Cranberry Oatmeal 14

Lunch 15

Salads 16
Almost Waldorf Salad (No Mayo) 17
Multi-Bean Salad 18
Scandinavian Potato Salad 19
Tasty Green Salad 20
Tomato, Cucumber and Cilantro Salad 21

Soups 22
Carrot & Pumpkin Soup 23
Split Pea Soup 24

Dinner 25

Slow Cooker Recipes 26
Autumn Harvest Stew 27
Black Bean Stew 28

Chickpea Curry With Spinach and Kale 29

Italian Bean Casserole 30

Vegetable and Lentil Stew 31

Oven Dinners 32

Cauliflower Cheese Casserole 33

Leek and Feta Quiche
With a Crispy Potato Crust 34

Lentil No-Meat Loaf 35

Oven-Baked Mexican Quinoa Casserole 36

Roasted Carrots and Parsnips 37

Roasted Baby Bok Choy 38

Easy Individual Pizzas 39

Skillet Dishes 40

Sautéed Red Cabbage 41

Vegetable Stir Fry 42

Desserts 43

Geoff's Easy Slow Cooker
Sugar-Free Rice Pudding 44

Peppered Strawberries 45

Mixed Fruit Cobbler 46

Sugar-Free Banana Bread 48

Raw Fruit Salad 50

Snacks 51

Frozen Grapes 52

Chewy Sugar-Free Granola Bars 53

Flour-less Sugarless Blueberry Muffins 54

Sugar-Free, Gluten-Free, Egg-Free,
Oil-Free Strawberry Muffins 55

Potato Skins 56

Raw Veggies and Dip 57

Geoff's Famous Hummus 58

Creamy Dill Hummus 59

Spicy Jalapeno Dill Hummus 60

Extras 61

Vegetable Broth 62

Bread Machine Rye Bread 63

Whole Wheat Sunflower Seed Bread 64

Easy Buttermilk Biscuits 65

Stir Fry Sauce #1 66

Stir Fry Sauce #2 67

Warm Horseradish Sauce 68

Roasted Garlic Salad Dressing 69

How to Roast Garlic 70

Adjust Your Own Recipes 71

Free Gift Now
All Our Books Free Later 72

Contact Us 73

About The Author 74

More books from Geezer Guide Publishing 75

This page deliberately left blank

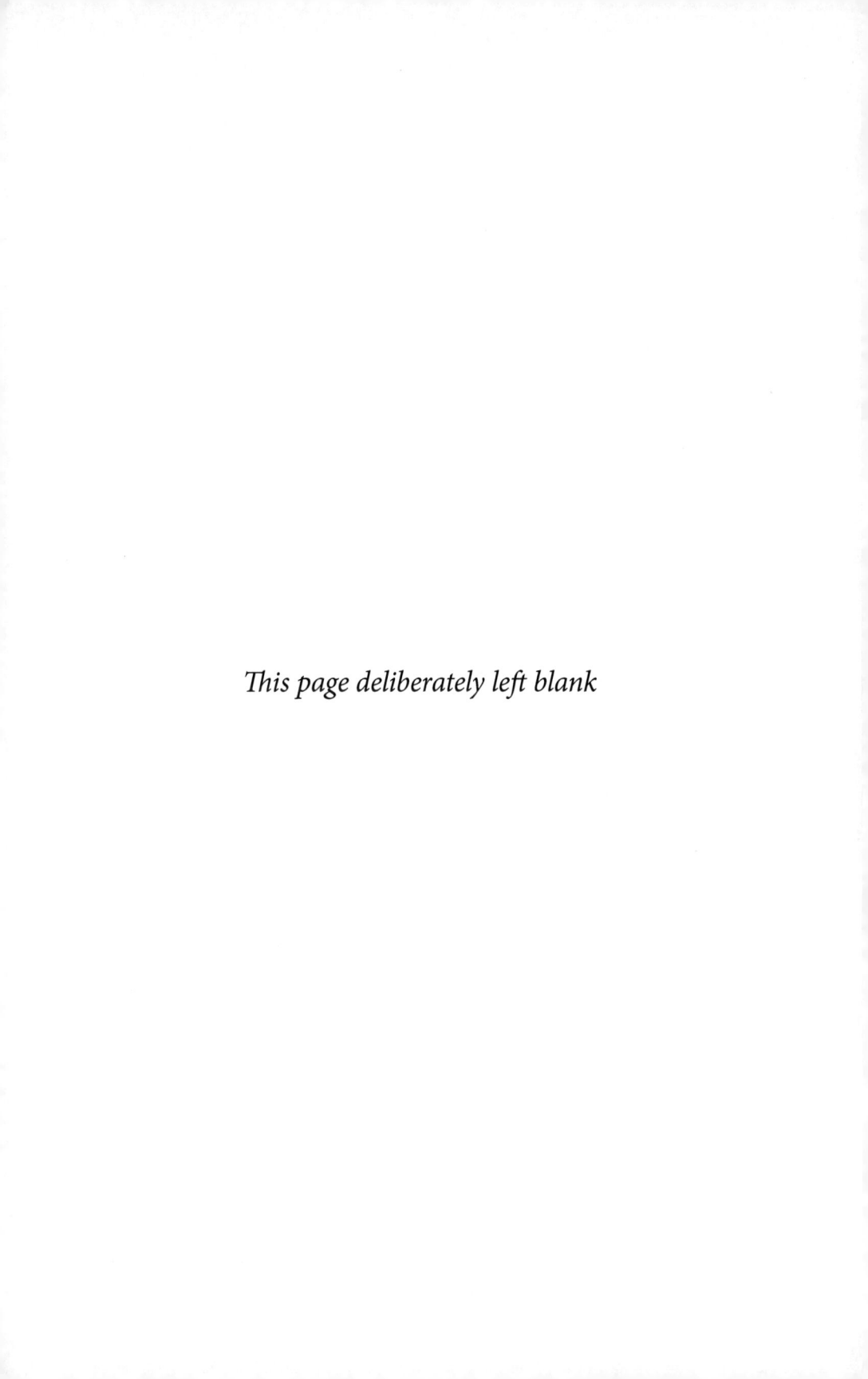

Foreword
Resetting Leptin Resistance

Leptin is the hormone responsible for regulating energy intake and energy expenditure. Simply put, when you have enough stored energy, leptin triggers satiety - it tells you you're full.

The problem with our modern, sugar-laden diet is that it can cause a serious imbalance in this hormone. The culprit has been identified as fructose. This is the same sugar found in fruit but without fruit's mitigating fibre. Regular table sugar is 50% glucose and 50% fructose, however, High Fructose Corn Syrup (HFCS), which is found in most soft drinks and juices, is 55% or more fructose. Other sweeteners, such as agave syrup, can be much higher

Fructose is naturally occurring in fruits, so should we stop eating fruits? The answer is a resounding NO! When we eat whole fruits, they also contain a lot of fiber which helps to mitigate the effects of the fructose.

Another key to resetting leptin resistance is to avoid any processed, packaged foods. In a lot of cases, fiber is sacrificed in order to extend shelf life. Also, many processed food manufactures have opted to use High Fructose Corn Syrup (HFCS) because it is cheaper and sweeter than regular sugar. Not only is that bad for us but it is most likely made from GMO corn.

This is a sugar-free cookbook so the recipes are perfect for anyone trying to reset their leptin response. However, just eating a sugar free diet won't reset your leptin levels, that requires the following:

Exercise

Go for a brisk 30 minute walk before breakfast and again before supper. By "brisk" we mean you need to get your heart rate up for most of the walk, then slow down for the last 5 minutes or so to get your heart rate back down again.

High Protein Breakfast

Have more protein and fewer carbohydrates for breakfast. Unfortunately, most modern breakfasts consist of hi-carb cereals or, even worse, sugar-loaded muffins or a pastry of some sort.

Even if you are vegetarian or vegan, it's still possible to have a high protein breakfast, like pancakes made with almond flour. As an example, see the Buckwheat and Almond Flour Blueberry Pancakes recipe in the Breakfast section of this book.

HAVE ONLY THREE MEALS A DAY

In order to effectively reset your leptin level, you need to restrict yourself to only three meals a day

APPROPRIATE PORTION SIZES

In our "super size" world, we are often presented with portion sizes much larger than are actually recommended or required. It's important to get back to normal portion sizes that are appropriate to your needs. Most of us tend to eat a lot more than we should, so it's important to learn about recommended portion sizes.

LONG BREAKS BETWEEN MEALS

Also, to effectively reset your lepton, it's important to leave at least 5 or 6 hours between meals. This allows your body to start using up reserves before your add more by eating again.

NO SNACKING

Most importantly, Don't Snack. Even the sugar-free snacks we have included in this book will derail your attempts to reset your leptin response.

If you eat between meals your body never gets a chance to use the energy from the last meal. In particular, don't eat after your evening meal and leave at least 12 hours between supper and breakfast.

Suggested additional sources for genuine information about leptin resistance:

BOOKS:

Sugar and the Evil Empire - the companion book to this cookbook

Fat Chance - by Dr. Robert Lustig

YOUTUBE VIDEOS WITH DR. ROBERT LUSTIG

Sugar - The Bitter Truth

Fat Chance: Fructose 2.0

Introduction

First Things First

We want to be very clear about the fact that when we say sugar-free that does NOT mean calorie-free. We have found that too many people are confused about this very important fact.

It is also important to note that calories are not necessarily a bad thing. We all need to consume a certain number of calories each day in order to survive. What is important is where those calories come from.

We all know that sugar supplies "empty" calories. What we often don't know is where sugar is lurking in our food. And, to make things worse, when most foods are processed, a lot of their nutrients, and their fiber, are removed. So we're hit with a kind of a double-whammy by losing the very things that can lessen the impact of sugar on our bodies.

Life In The Fast Lane

For most of us, life is run in the fast lane and fast, convenient foods have become the norm. But that's exactly the wrong thing to be fueling an active, fast-paced life. Most packaged and/or fast foods are devoid of the nutrients and micro-nutrients we need in order to survive and thrive in this fast-paced world.

That's right - we're setting ourselves up to fail, to get fat, to get sick and even worse.

Is There A Solution?

What's the solution to the need for fast food? We need to make our own.

As we learned in the book "Sugar and The Evil Empire", Big Food doesn't care about our health at all, they only care about their bottom line and satisfying their investors. They use every trick in the book, just like the tobacco companies did, in order to get us hooked and keep us coming back for more. They care more about things like shelf life than nutrition. They care more about getting us hooked so we'll buy more and more and more. Let's not ever fool ourselves that they have our best interests at heart, no matter what they say. We're smarter than that.

Making Our Own Fast Food

How fast can food be if we have to stop and make it ourselves? Well, with a little pre-planning, it's actually not that difficult. It will take some time but we can make our "fast food" ahead so it's ready when we don't have the time to prepare anything.

We can all find a few hours (or maybe even just minutes) to prepare some healthy fare, either in advance or with quick, healthy recipes.

USING A SLOW COOKER

There are several recipes in this book that make use of a slow cooker. This handy kitchen appliance makes it possible to time-shift the preparation and completion of meals. And, slow cookers are not just for dinner, either. Check out the breakfast recipes that can be started before retiring for the evening, allowing you to wake up to a fully cooked hot breakfast!

BUY ORGANIC WHEN POSSIBLE

Yes, organic can sometimes be expensive and most of us have a limited food budget. So what can we do?

Having all of our food organically grown is, of course, the ultimate goal. But that may be cost prohibitive for many of us. So, here's a few hints, cheats, if you will, on how to be as organic as possible.

We understand the difficulty of having access to organic produce. We, ourselves, live in a small town and have limited options.

THE DIRTY DOZEN

These foods are the most contaminated when being grown conventionally with all the herbicides, pesticides and chemical fertilizers.

When possible, purchase organically grown versions of these foods.

The Dirty Dozen (in order of most contamination) from http://www.davidsuzuki.org/what-you-can-do/queen-of-green/faqs/food/what-are-the-dirty-dozen-and-the-clean-fifteen/

- Apples
- Celery
- Sweet bell peppers
- Peaches
- Strawberries
- Nectarines
- Grapes
- Spinach
- Lettuce
- Cucumbers
- Blueberries
- Potatoes

The Clean Fifteen

When our budgets are limited we cannot always purchase organically grown foods. These items are the least contaminated even when conventionally grown.

The Clean Fifteen (in order of least contamination) from http://www.davidsuzuki.org/what-you-can-do/queen-of-green/faqs/food/what-are-the-dirty-dozen-and-the-clean-fifteen/

- Onions
- Sweet Corn
- Pineapples
- Avocado
- Cabbage
- Sweet peas
- Asparagus
- Mangoes
- Eggplant
- Kiwi
- Cantaloupe
- Sweet potatoes
- Grapefruit
- Watermelon
- Mushrooms

Supporting Our Local Farmers Markets

By supporting our local farmers markets we can do many good things. We can talk directly with the growers of our food to find out how our food is grown. It's much easier to find organic produce at your local farmers market.

But, not only that, we can support our local economy and support the smaller, family farms rather than Big Agriculture who are systematically destroying the traditional family farms.

It's a win-win - for us and for the local, family farms.

Growing Our Own Organic Produce

Not everyone has the time, space or ability to grow their own food. However, if we can, we certainly should.

Start small and build. Even if we only grow a few cherry tomatoes and some herbs in a pot on our kitchen counter, it's a start - a very good start.

Most Recipes In This Book Are Vegetarian and/or Vegan

You'll find, in this book, that most recipes are vegetarian or vegan. Why? Well, because after much research, that's the best, cleanest, way to eat.

We also can't condone the treatment of food animals. Did you know that animal cruelty laws do not apply to food animals? Well, they don't. And some of these animals live short, brutal lives.

But that's not the only reason. Besides being treated poorly, they are subjected to things like growth hormones and antibiotics. According to http://www.sustainabletable.org/257/antibiotics "Today, antibiotics are routinely fed to livestock, poultry, and fish on industrial farms to promote faster growth and to compensate for the unsanitary conditions in which they are raised. According to a new report by the FDA, approximately 80 percent of all antibiotics used in the United States are fed to farm animals."

The use of antibiotics and growth hormones is widespread in the USA, particularly in feedlot operations AKA CAFOs (**C**oncentrated **A**nimal **F**eeding **O**perations).

In Canada, according to Eat Right Ontario, "growth hormones are only given to beef cattle (and not dairy cattle). There are no growth hormones used in poultry or pork production". Eat Right Ontario also suggests picking organic options for both meat and vegetables in order to minimize any exposure to unwanted growth hormones or antibiotics.

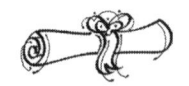

Breakfast

It's sad that sugary breakfast cereals have become the norm. There's so much more to love about breakfast and still be able to avoid the excess of sugar that seems to dominate the cereal aisle.

BUCKWHEAT PANCAKES

Servings: 8 (3 pancakes per serving) ❖ Calories per serving: 259

Yes, we can still have pancakes and have them sugar-free, too! Not only that, this can be one of the fast foods we have become so enamored with in our busy, busy lives. These pancakes can be cooked ahead, frozen and then reheated.

What could be easier than microwaving a few of these delicious pancakes for a quick breakfast on a busy day?

INGREDIENTS:

- 2 cups buckwheat flour, preferably organic
- 1 cup 7 grain cereal (or unbleached all-purpose flour)
- 3 cups non-dairy milk (like coconut, almond or rice)
- 2½ tablespoons baking powder
- 2 large eggs
- 4 tablespoons extra virgin olive oil

DIRECTIONS:

1. Pre-heat the oven to 170°F and place an oven-safe plate in the oven. This will be used to keep the pancakes warm as they are cooked.
2. In a large bowl, combine the buckwheat flour, multi-grain cereal (or all-purpose flour) and baking powder. Mix well.
3. In a large measuring cup, beat the eggs well. Then add the non-dairy milk and olive oil. Stir well.
4. Pour the liquid mixture into the dry mixture, stirring while pouring. Mix until everything is well combined but still a little lumpy. Do not over mix.
5. Coat a large skillet, or griddle, with some coconut or olive oil and heat over medium-high heat.
6. When the skillet is well heated, pour approximately ¼ to ⅓ cup of the pancake mixture into the skillet for each pancake. Depending on the size of the skillet you can probably cook about 2-4 pancakes at a time.
7. Cook until bubbles appear on the top of the batter and the bottom becomes a golden brown (approximately 1-2 minutes at the correct skillet temperature). Turn the pancakes and cook on the opposite side until golden brown (approximately 1 to 2 minutes).

    Note: Temperatures will vary from stove to stove but it should only take a few pancakes to get the hang of it.

8. As the pancakes are ready, transfer them to the plate in the warm oven and continue cooking pancakes until you have run out of batter.
9. Top with your choice of toppings - fruit, maple syrup, etc. Just be mindful of the nutrition and the calories of the toppings you choose.

Multi-Grain Hot Cereal

Servings: 8 ❖ Calories per serving: 305

Put this in your slow cooker just before heading off to bed, then it will be ready first thing in the morning. The ginger gives it a lovely flavor. You may want to add a non-dairy milk and a little more maple syrup to each serving. You can substitute honey for the maple syrup, if you like.

Ingredients:
- ½ cup brown basmati rice, rinsed
- ½ cup quinoa, rinsed
- ¼ cup flax seed, whole
- ¼ cup chia seeds
- 1 cup old fashioned oats
- 1 cup blueberries, fresh or frozen
- 1 teaspoon ground ginger
- 1 teaspoon sea salt
- ½ cup walnuts, chopped
- ¼ cup maple syrup
- 5 cups water

Directions:
1. Lightly oil the crock of your slow cooker.
2. Combine all of the ingredients in your slow cooker and stir to mix.
3. Set the slow cooker to low and cook for approximately 6 to 8 hours.
4. Serve warm directly from slow cooker.

Buckwheat and Almond Flour Blueberry Pancakes

Servings: 8 (3 pancakes per serving) ❖ Calories per serving: 316

Feeling a little more creative? This gluten-free pancake recipe also provides almost 10 grams of protein thanks to the almond flour. The blueberries are optional and you can substitute other fruits if you like or just leave the fruit out altogether.

These pancakes freeze well and can be reheated using a microwave or a toaster oven for a quick and easy meal.

Ingredients:

- 2 cups buckwheat flour, preferably organic
- 1 cup almond flour
- 2½ tablespoons baking powder
- 2 large eggs
- 3 cups almond milk, unsweetened
- 4 tablespoons olive oil
- 1 cup blueberries, fresh or frozen (optional)

DIRECTIONS:

1. Pre-heat the oven to 170°F and place an oven-safe plate in the oven. This will be used to keep the pancakes warm as they are cooked.
2. In a large bowl, combine the buckwheat flour, almond flour and baking powder. Mix well.
3. In a large measuring cup, beat the eggs well. Then add the almond milk and olive oil. Stir well.
4. Pour the liquid mixture into the dry mixture, stirring while pouring. Mix until everything is well combined but still a little lumpy. Do not over mix.
5. Gently fold in the blueberries, if using.
6. Coat a large skillet with some coconut or olive oil and heat over medium-high heat.
7. When the skillet is well heated, pour approximately ¼ to ⅓ cup of the pancake mixture into the skillet for each pancake. Depending on the size of the skillet you can probably cook about 2-4 pancakes at a time.
8. Cook until bubbles appear on the top of the batter and the bottom becomes a golden brown (approximately 1-2 minutes at the correct skillet temperature). Turn the pancakes and cook on the opposite side until golden brown (approximately 1 to 2 minutes).

Note: Temperatures will vary from stove to stove but it should only take a few pancakes to get the hang of it.

9. As the pancakes are ready, transfer them to the plate in the warm oven and continue cooking pancakes until you have run out of batter.
10. Top with your choice of toppings - fruit, maple syrup, etc. Just be mindful of the nutrition and the calories of the toppings you choose.

Vicky's Sugar-Free Granola
Servings: 16 ❖ Calories per serving: 371

This granola tastes a lot better, and is a lot better for you, than any of the commercial, sugar-laden cereals you'll find in the breakfast aisle. It is a staple in our household and we almost go into panic mode when we run out.

Yes, it is high calorie, but it's good for us. A serving of ½ cup, with a little non-dairy milk (almond milk, coconut milk, rice milk - all non-GMO, of course), is all that you need.

INGREDIENTS:

4 cups rolled oats, old fashioned, not quick or minute
½ cup chia seeds
½ cup oat bran
½ cup ground flax seed
½ cup sunflower seeds
½ cup almonds, chopped
½ cup walnuts, chopped
½ teaspoon sea salt
½ cup honey
½ cup maple syrup
⅓ cup coconut oil
2 teaspoons ground cinnamon
1½ teaspoons vanilla extract
1 cup raisins
6 Medjool dates, pitted and chopped
1 tablespoon almonds, finely ground

DIRECTIONS:

1. Pre-heat the oven to 325° F and lightly grease a large baking sheet.
2. Combine the oats, chia seeds, ground flax seeds, oat bran, sunflower seeds, almonds and walnuts in a large bowl.
3. In a small saucepan, mix together the salt, honey, maple syrup, coconut oil, cinnamon and vanilla. Over medium heat, bring the mixture to a boil and immediately remove from heat.
4. Pour the liquid mixture over the oat mixture and stir well to coat everything evenly. Then spread the mixture evenly on the greased baking sheet.
5. Bake at 325° F for 20 minutes, Remove from the oven and allow to cool.
6. While the granola is baking, chop up the Medjool dates and then toss them in the ground almonds to prevent them from sticking together. Once the oatmeal mixture has cooled, break it up and add the raisins and dates. Toss together to mix well.
7. Store the completed granola in an airtight container.

Note: We wish we could tell you how long it keeps in an airtight container, but it never lasts very long in our house.

Overnight Cranberry Oatmeal
Servings: 4 ❖ Calories per serving: 259

Start this vegan oatmeal recipe before bed and have it ready for breakfast the next morning. The prunes will add sweetness to the oatmeal so you may, or may not, want to add maple syrup as a garnish.

Ingredients:
   1 cup old fashioned oats
   1 cup cranberries, fresh or frozen

   Note: DO NOT use dried, sweetened cranberries as they often contain a lot of added sugar.

   1 cup prunes, chopped
   2 cups water
   2 cups non-dairy milk
   maple syrup, for garnish

Directions:
1. Lightly oil the crock of your slow cooker.
2. In the slow cooker, combine all the ingredients except the maple syrup. Stir gently and cover with the lid. Set the slower cook on low and cook for 7 to 8 hours.
3. Serve hot with a splash of maple syrup, if desired.

LUNCH

Lunches can often be challenging which is why we turn to the fast food industry so often to supply our midday meal. Most of the recipes here can be made ahead and packaged into meal-size servings that are easily transportable. Most workplaces now have some kind of kitchen with at least a fridge and a microwave.

> *Note: If you're planning to reheat food in a microwave, it's best to do it in glass, not plastic.*

SALADS

Salads make a great lunch. If you're pressed for time in the morning, make your salad the night before, package the dressing separately and put them together just before eating.

Almost Waldorf Salad (No Mayo)

Servings: 2 ❖ Calories per serving: 313

Waldorf salad is, of course, a classic. In this take we've eliminated the mayonnaise and replaced it with hummus. If you need to thin the hummus a bit, just add a little lemon juice and olive oil to achieve the desired consistency.

Note: There are several hummus recipes in the "Extras" section of this book. Commercially produced hummus may contain sugar and GMOs. If you choose a commercial product, read the label very carefully.

Ingredients:

- 1 medium red apple, cored and chopped
- 1 teaspoon lemon juice, freshly squeezed
- ½ cup walnuts, chopped
- ½ cup celery, sliced
- ½ cup seedless grapes, halved
- ¼ cup hummus
- sea salt, to taste
- black pepper, to taste
- 2-3 cups mixed baby greens

Directions:

1. Toss the chopped apple in the lemon juice to prevent browning.
2. In a large bowl, combine the chopped apple, walnuts, celery and grapes. Mix in the hummus and make sure everything is well coated.
3. Add salt and pepper to taste and serve over a bed of mixed greens.

Multi-Bean Salad
Servings: 10 ❖ Calories per serving: 271

Why settle for a three-bean salad? This is our favorite, make-from-scratch, multi-bean salad! It keeps well and makes a great addition to any lunch.

Ingredients:

1½ cups kidney beans, cooked
1½ cups chickpeas, cooked
1 cup baby lima beans, cooked
1 cup black beans, cooked
1½ cups green beans, cooked, straight cut
½ medium red onion, diced
2 stalks celery, diced
¼ medium green bell pepper, diced
¼ medium red bell pepper, diced
2 garlic cloves, pressed
½ cup extra virgin olive oil
½ cup white vinegar
¼ cup balsamic vinegar
½ cup pure honey
1½ teaspoons sea salt
1 teaspoon black pepper, freshly ground

Directions:

Note: All the beans in this recipe were cooked from dried beans with the exception, of course, for the green beans. They were cooked from fresh.

Note: You can substitute canned beans in the recipe if it's easier for you. Just be sure to rinse the canned beans very well to eliminate any unwanted salt.

1. In a large glass bowl, combine all the beans, red onion, celery, and peppers.

Note: you don't want to use metal bowls when using vinegar. You could use plastic but glass works much better.

2. In a large measuring cup, combine the olive oil, vinegars, honey, salt and pepper. Whisk well until ingredients are well combined.
3. Pour the oil and vinegar mixture over the bean mixture and stir well with a wooden spoon.
4. Cover the bean salad and refrigerate for at least 4 hours before serving. This allows all the flavors to blend and mature.

Scandinavian Potato Salad
Servings: 4 ❖ Calories per serving: 370

This is a lovely, and unusual, potato salad that can be made the night before. It also includes some canned salmon, so it's a complete lunch with a good amount of protein.

Ingredients:

- 1½ pounds small red potatoes, leave skins on
- ¾ cup sour cream (preferably organic)
- ¼ cup parsley, chopped
- ¼ cup dill pickles (no sugar added), chopped
- 2 tablespoons fresh dill, chopped
- ½ teaspoon horseradish
- ¼ teaspoon sea salt
- ¼ teaspoon black pepper, freshly ground
- ½ cup red onion, chopped
- 1 can red salmon, 7½ ounces

Directions:

1. Scrub the red potatoes well and leave whole. Place in a steamer and steam until they are just tender, about 20-25 minutes. Remove from steamer and allow them to cool completely. Then cut in half or into 4 wedges depending on the size of the potatoes.
2. In a large bowl, combine the sour cream, parsley, chopped pickles, dill, horseradish, salt and pepper. Whisk together until everything is well combined.
3. Add the potatoes, onion and salmon. Toss gently to ensure that everything is well combined and well coated.

Tasty Green Salad

Servings: 4 ❖ Calories per serving: 122

A quick and easy salad. If you grow you own greens, so much the better. If not, try to find the freshest ones available and use them right away.

Ingredients:

1 medium red apple, seeded and chopped
2 tablespoons extra virgin olive oil
¼ teaspoon fresh lemon peel, grated
1 tablespoon fresh lemon juice
2 teaspoons apple cider vinegar
2 teaspoons red onion, minced
1 teaspoon maple syrup
8 cups mixed greens, (romaine, arugula, spinach, kale, etc.)
freshly ground black pepper, to taste

Directions:

1. After chopping the apple, toss it in a little lemon juice to prevent browning.
2. Wash the greens, rinse well and spin or pat dry. Place them in a large salad bowl and set aside.
3. In a large measuring cup, whisk together the olive oil, lemon peel, lemon juice, vinegar, red onion and maple syrup. Then mix the apples into this dressing.
4. Gently pour the dressing over the mixed greens and toss to coat.
5. Grind the black pepper on the top, to taste, and serve immediately.

Note: If making the night before, place the dressing (including the chopped apple) in a separate container, apply to the greens and toss just before eating.

Tomato, Cucumber and Cilantro Salad

Servings: 4 ❖ Calories per serving: 61

This salad is tasty, filling and super-low in calories. It needs to be made ahead to allow the flavors to blend.

> *Note: Cilantro is one of those tastes that people either love or hate. There doesn't seem to be any middle ground. In our family, Vicky loves it, but Geoff hates it. So, Vicky gets this salad all to herself.*

Ingredients:

- 4 medium ripe tomatoes, cut in wedges
- 1 large English cucumber, sliced
- ½ medium red onion, chopped
- ½ medium green bell pepper, chopped
- 2 cloves garlic, minced
- ¼ cup fresh cilantro, chopped
- 2 tablespoons balsamic vinegar
- sea salt, to taste
- black pepper, freshly ground, to taste

Directions:

1. In a large bowl, combine all the ingredients and gently toss to coat.
2. Cover and refrigerate for at least ½ hour to allow the flavors to blend.
3. Serve on a bed of lettuce. Add more salt and pepper, if desired.

Soups

Soups can make for an easily portable lunch if you have access to a microwave at work. Be sure to package the soup up into individual servings so you can just grab and go. These soups will freeze well, too. So, you can just grab a serving from the freezer and let it defrost at work before heating it up.

Carrot & Pumpkin Soup

Servings: 8 ❖ Calories per serving: 236

This is a smooth, tasty, vegan soup that evokes the flavors of autumn. Make it ahead to let the flavors mature, then refrigerate or freeze.

Ingredients:

- 4 tablespoons extra virgin olive oil
- 1 large yellow onion, chopped
- 1 tablespoon ginger root, peeled and finely diced
- 6 cloves garlic, minced
- 6 cups vegetable broth
- 2 cups coconut milk
- 2 large carrots, peeled and chopped
- 4 cups pumpkin puree, or 1 30 oz. can
- 2 teaspoons pumpkin pie spice
- 1 teaspoon sea salt
- ½ teaspoon black pepper

Directions:

1. Heat olive oil in a large stock pot or dutch oven over medium heat.
2. Add the onion, ginger and garlic; sauté for 5-10 minutes.
3. Add the broth, water, carrots, pumpkin and pumpkin pie spice to the pot and heat until boiling.
4. Reduce the heat and simmer uncovered until the carrots are very tender, about 30 minutes.
5. Puree the soup in batches using a blender or a food processor.
6. Season with salt and pepper, to taste.

Split Pea Soup

Servings: 8 ❖ Calories per serving: 199

This tasty vegan soup cooks all day which helps blend the flavors. Let the slow cooker do all the work and then package up individual servings.

Ingredients:

- 2 cups split peas
- 4 medium carrots, chopped
- 2 cups cabbage, shredded
- 1 stalk celery, chopped
- 1 medium yellow onion, chopped
- 2 cloves garlic, minced
- 1 bay leaf
- 1 tablespoon salt
- ½ teaspoon pepper
- 6 cups vegetable broth, or water

Directions:

1. Lightly oil the crock of your slow cooker.
2. Layer ingredients in order listed, except for the vegetable broth, and don't stir it.
3. Gently pour the vegetable broth over the top, cover, set the slow cooker to low and cook for about 8 hours. The split peas should no longer be hard.
4. Remove the bay leaf and serve hot or package into individual servings and refrigerate or freeze.

DINNER

For busy families, trying to get a nutritious dinner on the table, quickly, can be a major challenge. In a lot of these recipes we'll employ a slow cooker. To make things even easier, cut up and measure all the ingredients the night before so they can be easily added to the slow cooker in the morning before leaving for work and school.

SLOW COOKER RECIPES

We've always like to use slow cookers when possible, particularly if we have a busy day planned. It's so nice to get home have dinner ready with little to no fuss.

A lot of different meals lend themselves to this kind of cooking and once you get used to using a slow cooker, you'll even find yourself putting together a meal without the aid of a recipe.

Autumn Harvest Stew

Servings: 6 ❖ Calories per serving: 214

This is one of our favorite recipes. The combination of the root vegetables, cabbage, caraway and apples makes for an interesting and tasty stew. You can serve this with potatoes, yams or rice. This recipe is high fiber, high nutrients and very low calorie making it a great addition to any weight loss program. In addition to all that, it's vegan too!

Ingredients:

- ¾ cup yellow split peas
- ½ head cabbage, sliced
- 3 medium carrots, chunked
- 3 medium parsnips, chunked
- 1 large yellow onion, sliced
- 1 apple, cored and sliced
- 4 cups vegetable broth
- ½ cup unsweetened apple sauce
- 1 teaspoon dried basil
- 1 ½ teaspoons caraway seed
- 1 teaspoon kosher salt
- ½ teaspoon black pepper, freshly ground

Directions:

1. Place all the ingredients in the slow cooker and stir to combine.
2. Set the slow cooker on low for 8-10 hours.
3. Remove 1½ to 2 cups of the stew and puree in a blender, then return the puree to the stew and stir well. Doing this helps thicken the stew.
4. Serve immediately.
5. Any leftovers can be frozen for future use.

Black Bean Stew

Servings: 4 ❖ Calories per serving: 246

For this vegan recipe we used frozen tomatoes and zucchini from our garden. We have always said, the best way to get organic produce is to grow it yourself. If you're using vegetables you've frozen yourself, be sure to let them thaw in a colander and catch any of the water that runs off. Save the water to add to your homemade vegetable broth. Thawing the veggies this way will make them a little firmer and they'll stand up in the stew better.

Naturally, this recipe works just fine with fresh vegetables, too.

Ingredients:

- 6 tomatoes, chopped
- 1 small zucchini, chopped
- 1 medium yellow onion, chopped
- 1 jalapeno, chopped
- 2 stalks celery, sliced
- ¼ cup tomato paste
- ¼ cup sun dried tomatoes, chopped
- 3 tablespoons taco seasoning
- ½ cup corn
- 2 cups black beans, home cooked or canned, drained and rinsed
- 1 cup kale, packed, chopped
- 1 teaspoon pepper

Directions:

1. Combined all the ingredients in the slow cooker except the kale. Stir well.
2. Set the slow cooker on low for 6-8 hours.
3. Add the kale and stir well. Turn the slow cooker to high for about 30 minutes, then reduce to low for another 30 minutes.
4. Serve over brown rice.

Chickpea Curry With Spinach and Kale

Servings: 4 ❖ Calories per serving: 263

This East Indian-inspired vegan recipe combines some wonderful flavors and is high in nutrients and anti-oxidants. The kale and spinach also add calcium to the mix.

Ingredients:

- 2 medium yellow onions, diced
- 2 cloves garlic, minced
- 2 teaspoons fresh ginger, minced
- 1 teaspoon cumin seeds, whole
- 1 teaspoon ground cumin
- 1 teaspoon ground coriander
- ½ teaspoon garam masala
- ½ teaspoon turmeric
- ½ teaspoon sea salt
- 28 ounces diced tomatoes, canned, with juice
- 2 cups chickpeas, home cooked or canned
- 2 tablespoons tomato paste
- 2 cups kale, stem removed and chopped
- 2 cups baby spinach, chopped

Directions:

1. Lightly oil the crock of your slow cooker.
2. Combine all of the ingredients in the slow cooker, with the exception of the kale and spinach. Stir well.
3. Cover the slow cooker with the lid and set to low. Cook for approximately 6-7 hours.
4. Just before it is done, turn the slow cooker to high, add the kale and spinach, and cook for another 20 minutes.
5. Serve hot with rice or cous cous.

Italian Bean Casserole

Servings: 6 ❖ Calories per serving: 413

You can use any kind of pasta you choose for this vegan recipe. We used elbow macaroni. If you use spaghetti or some other long noodle, be sure to break it up into smaller pieces. This nutritious meal is high in fiber, thanks to the beans, and has no added fat.

Note: You can use canned beans in the recipe, just be sure to rinse them well to remove any unwanted salt. Substitute a 19 ounce can of Great Northern Beans and a 19 ounce can of small red beans (or kidney beans) for the dried beans and eliminate the 5 cups of cold water as that would have been used to soak the dried beans.

Ingredients

- 1 cup great Northern Beans, dry
- 1 cup small red beans, dry
- 5 cups cold water
- 28 ounces diced tomatoes, canned
- 1 medium yellow onion, chopped
- 1 stalk celery, chopped
- 4 cups vegetable broth
- 3 cloves garlic, minced
- 1 tablespoon Italian seasoning
- ½ teaspoon black pepper, freshly ground
- 1½ teaspoons sea salt
- 1 medium zucchini, chopped
- 8 ounces pasta, your choice

Directions:

1. In a large pot, combine the dry beans with approximately 5 cups of cold water. Bring the beans to a boil, reduce the heat and simmer for 2 minutes. Remove from the heat and let sit, covered, for 1 hour. Then drain and rinse the beans. OR skip this step and used canned beans as detailed above.
2. Add all the ingredients, with the exception of the zucchini and pasta, to your slow cooker. Stir well to combine. Set the slow cooker to low.
3. Cook on low for approximately 8-9 hours, then increase to high and add the zucchini and pasta. Cook for an additional hour on high. Pasta should be tender and the zucchini should be cooked.
4. Serve hot.

Note: This casserole freezes well.

Vegetable and Lentil Stew

Servings: 8 ❖ Calories per serving: 158

In this recipe we employed some tomatoes from our garden that we had frozen the previous season. We defrosted them slightly and coarsely chopped them. The vegetable broth was homemade from boiling any leftover veggies and peelings. You can substitute canned tomatoes and a commercial vegetable broth if you like - just try to make sure that you're getting low sodium and sugar-free versions.

And, yes, you guessed it - this recipe is vegan, too.

Ingredients:

- 1 cup lentils, green or brown
- 1 large yellow onion, chopped
- 2 cloves garlic, chopped
- ½ head cauliflower, broken into florets
- ¼ cup pearl barley
- 2 medium carrots, cut into chunks
- 2 stalks celery, sliced
- 1½ cups tomatoes, chopped
- 1 tablespoon herbes de Provence
- 1 bay leaf
- 1½ teaspoons sea salt
- 1 teaspoon black pepper, freshly ground
- 4 cups vegetable broth
- 2 cups kale, chopped (or substitute fresh baby spinach)

Directions:

1. Combine all ingredients in a slow cooker, with the exception of the kale (or baby spinach) and stir well.
2. Turn slow cooker to low and cook for 6-8 hours.
3. Turn slow cooker to high, add the kale (or baby spinach) and cook for an additional 30 minutes.
4. Stir well. Remove 1½ to 2 cups of the stew and puree it in a blender. Return the pureed stew to the slow cooker and stir well. This will help thicken the stew.
5. Serve immediately.

OVEN DINNERS

Preparing a meal ahead of time and then just popping it in the oven can be quite a time saver, too. Making extras gives you the option of reheating any leftovers for another meal.

Cauliflower Cheese Casserole

Servings: 4 ❖ Calories per serving: 588

This dish can be served as the main meal or as a side dish depending on the size of the serving. This recipe contains dairy - whole milk and cheddar cheese.

Ingredients:

- 1 head cauliflower, cut into florets
- 4 large russet potatoes, cut into large chunks
- 1 yellow onion, sliced
- 4 tablespoons butter
- 4 tablespoons flour
- ½ teaspoon dry mustard
- ¼ teaspoon black pepper, freshly ground
- 1½ cups whole milk
- 1½ cups sharp Cheddar cheese, shredded, divided

Directions:

1. Pre-heat the oven to 350°F.
2. Grease a 9 inch x 13 inch glass baking dish and arrange the cauliflower florets, potato chunks and sliced onion evenly in the dish. Set aside.
3. In a medium sauce, over medium heat, melt the butter. With a wooden spoon, slowly mix in the flour, dry mustard and pepper to create a roux. Once the roux has browned slightly, slowly stir in the whole milk and continue cooking until mixture begins to thicken. Add in 1 cup of the shredded cheese and continue stirring until the cheese has melted and the sauce is smooth. Remove the saucepan from the heat.
4. Evenly pour the cheese sauce over the vegetables in the baking dish and sprinkle the remaining ½ cup of shredded cheese over the top.
5. Bake at 350°F for about one hour or until the vegetables are cooked through and the cheese sauce is bubbly and has started to brown.
6. Remove the casserole from the oven and allow to cool, for about 5 minutes, on a wire rack before serving.

Leek and Feta Quiche
With a Crispy Potato Crust
Servings: 6 ❖ Calories per serving: 336

This recipe can be a little fiddly but is well worth it. It also includes dairy, eggs and some bacon. The bacon is optional and we have had great results without it.

Ingredients:

- 2 medium potatoes, scrubbed and thinly sliced
- 2 tablespoons butter, melted
- 2 slices bacon (optional)
- 1 cup leeks, cleaned and thinly sliced
- 3 eggs
- 1 cup cream
- 2 tablespoons fresh thyme, chopped
- ¼ teaspoon sea salt
- ¼ teaspoon black pepper, freshly ground
- 4 ounces feta cheese
- 2 green onions, sliced

Directions:

1. Pre-heat the oven to 375°F. Lightly grease a 9 inch pie plate.
2. Arrange a layer potato slices concentrically in the pie plate, starting from the outside working in and overlapping slightly. Brush the potatoes with the melted butter. Repeat to make a second layer and brush the second layer with the melted butter.
3. Bake the potato crust at 375°F for 15 minutes. Then remove from oven and cool on a wire rack.
4. While the potato crust is baking, in a medium skillet, cook the bacon until very crisp. Transfer the bacon to some paper towel to drain. Then remove the excess fat in the skillet leaving behind about a teaspoon of bacon grease (If you're not using the bacon, just add a teaspoon of butter to the pan). In the remaining grease cook the leek until softened, about 5 minutes. Remove the skillet from the heat and stir in the fresh thyme, salt and pepper.
5. Evenly sprinkle the leek mixture over the potato crust. Crumble the bacon (if using) and sprinkle it evenly over the leek mixture. Sprinkle the crumbled feta cheese on top of that.
6. In a small bowl, combine the eggs and cream and whisk well. Pour it overtop of everything in the pie plate.
7. Bake the quiche at 375°F for about 35 minutes or until it has puffed up and the egg mixture is completely set.
8. Remove from the oven and cool on a wire rack for about 10 minutes before slicing and serving.

Lentil No-Meat Loaf

Servings: 6 ❖ Calories per serving: 300

This is one of our favorite vegan dishes and we have it often. You can use either red or green lentils. Using red lentils will give the loaf a finer texture, using green ones will give it a coarser, "meatier" texture.

Ingredients:

- 2 cups water
- 1 teaspoon sea salt
- 1 cup lentils
- 1 small yellow onion, diced
- 1 stalk celery, minced
- 1 cup quick cooking oats
- 2 large eggs, beaten
- ½ cup tomato paste
- ¼ cup water
- ½ cup nutritional yeast
- 1 clove garlic, minced
- 1 teaspoon oregano, dried
- 1 tablespoon parsley, fresh, minced
- 1 teaspoon sea salt
- ½ teaspoon black pepper, freshly ground

Directions:

1. Pre-heat the oven to 350°F and lightly oil a glass loaf pan.
2. In a medium saucepan, boil the water and add the salt. Add the lentils, reduce the heat and put a cover on the pot. Cook for 30 minutes, until soft. Remove from heat and allow them to cool completely.
3. In a large bowl, mix together the cooled lentils, diced onion, diced celery and oats. Mixed well.
4. Add the tomato paste, water, nutritional yeast, garlic and spices.
5. Place the mixed in the oiled loaf pan and pat down.
6. Bake at 350°F for 45 minutes, until the top is well browned. Allow the loaf to cool for 10 minutes on a wire rack before slicing.

Oven-Baked Mexican Quinoa Casserole

Servings: 4 ❖ Calories per serving: 430

We're big fans of casseroles and Mexican food, so this gives us the best of both worlds. Although the nutritional yeast in this vegan recipe is optional, it helps impart a "cheesy" flavor to the dish.

Ingredients:

- 1 tablespoon olive oil
- 1 onion, chopped
- 2 clove garlic, minced
- 1 cup quinoa, rinsed
- 28 ounces diced tomatoes, can with liquid
- 1 cup water
- 2 tablespoons nutritional yeast, optional
- 1 tablespoon tomato paste
- 1 teaspoon cumin
- 1 teaspoon oregano
- 1 teaspoon chili powder, or more, to taste (we add up to a tablespoon depending on the strength of the chili powder)
- 1½ teaspoons sea salt
- ½ teaspoon black pepper, freshly ground
- 2 cups kidney beans, rinsed and drained
- 1 cup corn, fresh or frozen
- 3 cups baby spinach, chopped

Directions:

1. Pre-heat oven to 350°F. Lightly oil a 3-quart, oven-safe casserole dish.
2. In a medium skillet, over medium-high heat, heat the 1 tablespoon of olive oil and add the onion and garlic. Sauté until translucent, about 5 minutes and transfer to the casserole dish.
3. Add the quinoa, diced tomatoes (with juice), water, nutritional yeast, tomato paste, spices, salt and pepper. Stir well.
4. Cover the casserole, place in oven and bake for 30 minutes.
5. Carefully remove the casserole from oven and stir in the drained drained beans and corn. If the mixture looks dry, add a half cup of water.
6. Cover the casserole and return to the oven for another 30 minutes.
7. Carefully remove the casserole from oven and stir in the baby spinach, allowing it to wilt.
8. Serve immediately.

Roasted Carrots and Parsnips
Servings: 4 ❖ Calories per serving: 176

We are both big fans of carrots and parsnips - particularly roasted. This recipe works just fine without the addition of the maple syrup, but if you'd like a little sweeter taste, and a bit more of a glaze, then go ahead and add it. This makes a fine side dish for the Lentil "No-Meat" Loaf.

Ingredients:
- 4 large carrots
- 4 medium parsnips
- 1 tablespoons coconut oil
- 1 teaspoon coarse sea salt
- ½ teaspoon black pepper, freshly ground
- 1 tablespoon herbes de Provence
- 1 tablespoons maple syrup, optional

Directions:
1. Peel the carrots and parsnips, cut in half and then quarter, lengthwise. Place in medium bowl.
2. Pre-heat oven to 400°F.
3. Melt the coconut oil in the microwave and drizzle over carrots and parsnips. Add the salt, pepper, herbs de Provence and maple syrup. Toss well making sure the carrots and parsnips are well coated.
4. Spread the coated carrots and parsnips on the lightly greased baking sheet, in a single layer.
5. Bake at 400°F for 20-30 minutes or until soft and nicely browned.
6. Remove from oven and serve immediately.

Roasted Baby Bok Choy

Servings: 2 ❖ Calories per serving: 235

Normally we would use bok choy in a Chinese recipe, like a stir fry, but roasting it this way makes for an unusual and tasty side dish.

INGREDIENTS:
- 3 medium heads baby bok choy
- 2 tablespoons extra virgin olive oil
- 1 tablespoon balsamic vinegar
- 2 tablespoons maple syrup
- 1 teaspoon crushed red pepper flakes

DIRECTIONS:
1. Pre-heat the oven to 400°F.
2. Cut the baby bok choy in half, lengthwise, and wash and dry thoroughly.
3. In a glass measuring cup, mix together the oil, vinegar, maple syrup and red pepper flakes until well combined.
4. Place the bok choy is a shallow bowl and drizzle the oil and vinegar mixture over top. Then toss well to make sure the bok choy is well coated.
5. Transfer the coated bok choy to a greased, rectangular baking dish. Arrange the bok choy cut side up and do not overlap.
6. Bake at 400°F. for 10 minutes. Remove from oven and turn the bok choy cut side down. Return to oven and bake for another 10 minutes. The edges of the bok choy leaves will be wilted and, possibly, slightly blackened.
7. Remove from oven and serve immediately.

Easy Individual Pizzas
Servings: 2 ❖ Calories per serving: 358

Homemade pizza is usually a Friday night treat at our house. Frequently we make our own pizza dough, but this recipe uses flour tortillas and is super easy to make. Instead of using commercially made pizza sauce, just use canned tomato paste and add the spices separately. Check the ingredients on cans of tomato paste - most list only one ingredient - tomatoes. Pass on the tomato pastes that already have herbs added. Often those ones will also have added salt.

Note: When choosing the tortillas, look for ones that only have 4 or 5 ingredients - like flour, water, salt, etc. - names we can recognize and pronounce.

Ingredients:
- 2 10" flour tortillas
- 2 tablespoons tomato paste
- 2 teaspoons Italian spice
- 1 small tomato, thinly sliced
- 4 black olives, thinly sliced
- ¼ medium yellow onion, thinly sliced
- ¼ medium sweet bell pepper, thinly sliced
- 2 large mushrooms, thinly sliced
- 2 ounces mozzarella cheese, shredded

Directions:
1. Pre-heat the oven to 375°F and lightly grease a baking sheet.
2. Place the two tortillas on the baking sheet and bake for 3 minutes each side, then remove from oven and allow to cool. They should be slightly brown and just a little crisp.
3. On each tortilla, spread 1 tablespoon of tomato paste. Then split all of the remaining ingredients between each pizza (tortilla), ending with the mushrooms and then the shredded cheese.
4. Return the pizzas to the oven and bake at 375°F for approximately 10 to 15 minutes or until the cheese is melted and bubbly.
5. Remove from oven and transfer the pizzas to a cutting board. Allow to cool for a couple of minutes and then slice each pizza into four wedges using a pizza cutting wheel or a sharp knife.

SKILLET DISHES

Skillet dishes can be quick, easy and tasty. Here's a few that definitely fall into the category.

Sautéed Red Cabbage

Servings: 4 ❖ Calories per serving: 192

This is a surprisingly quick dish to prepare. It's a tasty side dish for just about any meal. And it's vegan, too.

Ingredients:

- 2 tablespoons coconut oil
- 1 small yellow onion, sliced
- 1 apple, chopped
- ½ head red cabbage, sliced
- ⅓ cup apple cider vinegar with "the mother"
- 1 tablespoon dijon mustard
- 2 tablespoons maple syrup
- sea salt, to taste
- black pepper, to taste
- 1 tablespoon caraway seeds
- ¼ cup raisins

Directions:

1. In a large skillet, over medium-high heat, melt the coconut oil and heat well.
2. Add the onion and sauté for 2-3 minutes.
3. Add the apple, cabbage, vinegar, mustard and maple syrup. Stir well and sauté for 4-5 minutes.
4. Salt and pepper to taste. Add the caraway seeds and raisins. Stir well.
5. Cover, reduce heat and simmer for 5 minutes.
6. Serve immediately.

Vegetable Stir Fry

Servings: 4 ❖ Calories per serving: 117
(excluding the stir fry sauce)

With all these veggies, this recipe makes for a satisfying and filling meal. Whichever version of the stir fry sauce is chosen, it's still a very low calorie option. Pair it with some organic brown rice. And, for those who eat meat, add 1-2 cups of pre-cooked chicken, pork or beef to the recipe just before it is done and cook only long enough to heat the meat through.

Ingredients:

1 teaspoon olive oil
1 medium yellow onion, halved and sliced
4 cloves garlic, minced
½ inch fresh ginger, piece, minced
2 medium carrots, cut into matchsticks
2 stalks celery, sliced
¼ medium cabbage, sliced
1 cup broccoli, chopped
½ large green bell pepper, chopped
½ large red bell pepper, chopped
1 cup sugar snap peas
1 medium zucchini, halved and sliced
6 mushrooms, sliced
1 cup sugar-free stir fry sauce (see two sugar-free sauce recipes in the Extras Section)

Directions:

1. Over medium-high heat, heat the oil in a large wok or deep frying pan.
2. Add the garlic and ginger and cook for a minute or two.
3. Add the onion, carrots and celery and stir fry for 4 to 5 minutes, then add the cabbage and the broccoli and stir fry for another 3 to 4 minutes.
4. Add all of the stir fry sauce and mix well. Cover and cook for 5 minutes.
5. Add the zucchini, peppers, mushrooms and sugar snap peas, stir and cover. Continue to cook for another 4-5 minutes.
6. Remove from heat and serve over rice.

DESSERTS

Sugar-free desserts are not that uncommon but a lot of them resort to artificial sweeteners to provide that sweet taste we all crave. We have not only eliminated the sugar but you won't find any artificial sweeteners in these recipes either.

Just another reminder, though. Sugar-free desserts are NOT calorie-free desserts. We still need to exercise control when indulging in any desserts. Sorry.

Geoff's Easy Slow Cooker Sugar-Free Rice Pudding

Servings: 16 ❖ Calories per serving: 133

Geoff's the rice pudding guru in our house and he's come up with a sugar-free winner here. This recipe makes a very dense rice pudding, (the way we like it). If you'd like it to be creamier, cut back on the rice a bit or add more milk.

Ingredients:

- 1 cup pearl rice
- 8 cups coconut/almond milk
- 2 teaspoons vanilla
- ¼ teaspoon salt
- 1 cup dates, chopped
- 1 cup golden raisins

Directions:

1. Add the rice, coconut/almond milk, vanilla, salt and dates to the slow cooker and stir well to combine.
2. Set slow cooker to high for the first hour and then reduce to low for another 3 hours.
3. 10 minutes before serving, add the golden raisins, stir to combine and replace the lid to make sure the raisins get warmed through.

Peppered Strawberries
Servings: 4 ❖ Calories per serving: 117

This is a wonderfully versatile recipe using strawberries - a favorite super food. You can serve this recipe, as-is, as either a dessert or an appetizer. You can also add these peppered strawberries to a salad as a colorful addition and an amazing taste experience. Or use them as a topping for your favorite dessert. The possibilities are endless - and delicious!

INGREDIENTS:

- 1 pound fresh strawberries, rinsed and patted dry
- ¼ cup balsamic vinegar
- ¼ cup honey
- 2 teaspoons black pepper, freshly ground

DIRECTIONS:

1. Hull and quarter the strawberries and place them in a glass bowl.
2. In a glass measuring bowl, whisk together the vinegar and honey until they are completely incorporated.
3. Pour the vinegar and honey mixture over the strawberries and toss to coat evenly.
4. Grind the black pepper over the strawberries and toss again.
5. Serve or refrigerate immediately.

Mixed Fruit Cobbler

Servings: 8 ❖ Calories per serving: 192

Traditionally made fruit cobbler is often loaded with sugar. In this recipe we've replaced the sugar in the fruit mixture with finely chopped Medjool dates. We've also replaced the sugar in the topping with unsweetened applesauce. And, this recipe has the added convenience of being made in a slow cooker!

Either fresh or frozen fruit works well in this recipe. When purchasing frozen fruit make sure it has no sugar added, or just buy extra fruit when it is in season and freeze it yourself. If you are unable to find fresh red currants, you can substitute blueberries.

Ingredients:

Fruit Filling

- 3 cups peaches, 3-4 medium peaches, pitted and sliced
- 2 cups golden plums, 14-16 small plums, pitted and sliced
- 1 cup red currants, fresh
- 6 medjool dates, finely chopped
- 4½ teaspoons cornstarch
- 1½ teaspoons lemon juice, fresh
- 1 teaspoon vanilla

Batter

- 1 cup whole wheat flour
- 1 teaspoons baking powder
- ½ teaspoon baking soda
- 2 tablespoons flax seed, ground
- ⅔ cup applesauce, unsweetened
- 1 tablespoon olive oil
- 1 teaspoon vanilla
- 2 tablespoons almond milk

DIRECTIONS:

1. Lightly oil the crock of your slow cooker.
2. Fruit Filling: In a large bowl, combine the peaches, plums, currants (or blueberries), sugar, cornstarch, lemon juice and vanilla extract. Toss to mix well. Spoon into the slow cooker.
3. Batter: In a large bowl, combine the first five ingredients (the dry ingredients) and mix well. Make a well in the center of the flour mixture and add the applesauce, oil, vanilla and almond milk. Stir well to create a smooth batter. Gently pour the batter over the fruit mixture.
4. Place the lid on the slow cooker and turn to High setting. Cook for about 4 hours. The topping should be fully cooked and the fruit filling should be bubbly.
5. Turn off the slow cooker, remove the lid and allow the cobbler to cool for 15 minutes before serving.

Sugar-Free Banana Bread

Servings: 20 (10 slices per loaf) ❖ Calories per serving: 156

Not only is there no refined sugar in this recipe, there's not even any honey or maple syrup. The sweetness is provided by the dates, prunes and bananas. Using dried fruits and bananas not only adds sweetness but also lots of fiber, vitamins and nutrients that you wouldn't get from sugar. The calorie count is also pretty reasonable for something like this. So enjoy!

Ingredients:

generous ½ cup dates, chopped
generous ½ cup prunes, chopped
1 cup water
½ cup unsweetened apple sauce
3 eggs
1 teaspoon vanilla
1 cup walnuts, chopped, optional
1 cup unbleached all-purpose flour
½ cup whole wheat flour
1 cups rolled oats
¼ cup flax seed meal
¼ cup oat bran
2½ teaspoons baking soda
¼ teaspoon salt
5 bananas, mashed

Directions:

1. In a small saucepan, combine the chopped dates and prunes with the water. Over medium heat, bring the mixture to a boil, reduce heat and continue to boil for 5 minutes. Allow the mixture to cool slightly and add the apple sauce. Mix well and pour into a large bowl.

   Note: *watch the saucepan very closely. This kind of mixture can boil over and burn very quickly. Be sure to reduce the heat so it just stays at a boil.*

2. Pre-heat the oven to 350°F and lightly oil two 8-inch x 4-inch loaf pans.
3. In a small bowl, beat the eggs well. Then add the vanilla and nuts, mix well. Add the egg mixture to the cooled prune and date mixture. Mix until everything is well combined.
4. In a medium bowl, mix together the all purpose flour, whole wheat flour, oats, bran, flax meal, baking soda and salt. Add this to the fruit and nut mixture and mix well.
5. Mash the bananas well and fold them into the batter, just until everything is combined. Do not over mix.

   Hint: *the easiest way we've found to mash bananas is to put them in a bowl and use a pastry blender to mash them.*

6. Pour the batter into the greased 8 inch x 4 inch baking loaf pans and bake at 350°F for 35-40 minutes or until browned and a toothpick inserted in the center comes out clean.
7. Remove from the oven and cool for at least 10 minutes on a wire rack. Remove the banana bread from the loaf pans and allow to cool completely on a wire rack.

Raw Fruit Salad

Servings: 12 ❖ Calories per serving: 126

We love fresh fruit - love it! This is probably our best "How Many Super Foods Can You Stuff In A Recipe" recipe. Use this for breakfast or as a dessert. Enjoy! And - don't leave out the pepper. It really enhances all the tastes and you won't taste the pepper itself at all - really.

Ingredients:

- 1 cup strawberries, sliced
- ½ cup raspberries
- ½ cup blueberries
- 1 kiwi, peeled and sliced
- 1 nectarine, pitted and sliced
- 1 sweet orange, peeled and chopped
- ½ cup pomegranate seeds
- 1 small pear, seeded and chopped
- 1 small apple, seeded
- ½ cup fresh pineapple chunks
- 1 teaspoon black pepper, freshly ground
- ½ cup almonds, chopped
- ½ cup walnuts, chopped
- ½ cup coconut meat, freshly grated, optional

Directions:

1. Carefully rinse and dry all the fruit.
2. In a large bowl, combine all of the ingredients with the exception of the nuts and the coconut (if using).
3. Toss the ingredients gently to mix well. Cover and refrigerate for at least one hour before serving to allow the flavors to mix and a natural juice to form.
4. Just before serving, add the nuts and the coconut.

Note: you may just want to sprinkle the nuts and coconut on top of each serving.

SNACKS

Processed snack foods are one of the places that sugar likes to hide, not to mention GMOs (**G**enetically **M**odified **O**rganism), added salt, preservatives, etc. It's a huge industry and the Big Food corporations know what they're doing when they manipulate the formulation of their products to make them irresistible. Don't let them hook you. Make your own convenient, healthy snacks and tell Big Food to take a hike!

For the full truth on sugar, how it is poisoning us and how Big Food corporations are profiting read "Sugar and the Evil Empire"

Just a reminder that if you are trying to reset your leptin response you must resist the temptation to eat between meals. Even sugar-free snacks will sabotage your efforts.

But there is no reason you can't try some of these "snacks" for breakfast or lunch.

FROZEN GRAPES

Servings: That will depend on the number of grapes we eat.

Calories per serving: 1 cup of seedless grapes is about 110 calories.

Okay, it just doesn't get any easier, or more delicious, than this. How many recipes are there that have only ONE ingredient and incredibly simple directions? And, yes, we'll be getting fructose from the snack. After all, it is fruit. However, we'll also be getting it in its natural form along with the fiber - just as nature intended.

INGREDIENTS:

1 bunch green seedless grapes (or more, or less - your choice)

DIRECTIONS:

1. Wash the grapes and pat them dry.
2. Remove the grapes from the stalk and, in a single layer, place them on a baking sheet lined with wax paper.
3. Place them in the freezer for several hours.
4. Repackage individually frozen grapes in resealable plastic bags and place them back in freezer for convenient snacking.

Chewy Sugar-Free Granola Bars

Servings: 16 ❖ Calories per serving: 237

This sugar-free, no-bake recipe makes lovely, chewy granola bars. You can alter the add-ins (sunflower seeds, raisins, etc.) so long as the total equals one cup, so be sure to experiment to get the type and taste you want.

Note: Don't go overboard on these, even though they are really tasty. Like we said before - sugar-free does NOT mean calorie free. And, at 237 calories per bar, these should be reserved for a special treat.

Ingredients:

½ cup natural peanut butter, smooth or chunky
⅓ cup honey
¼ cup coconut oil
1 cup old fashioned oats
¼ cup sunflower seeds
¼ cup raisins
¼ cup pepitas (pumpkin seeds)
¼ cup chia seeds

Directions

1. Lightly grease an 8 inch x 8 inch glass baking dish and set aside.
2. In a medium saucepan, combine the peanut butter, honey and coconut oil. Heat over medium-low heat and stir until all ingredients are melted and well combined.
3. Remove the saucepan from the heat and add in the remaining ingredients. Stir well with a wooden spoon and make sure all ingredients are well mixed.
4. Pour the mixture into the greased baking dish, using a silicone spatula to get all of the mixture out of the saucepan and to press the mixture firmly into the baking dish.
5. Chill for at least two hours. Cut the mixture into 16 equal squares. Gently remove them from the baking dish and wrap individually with plastic wrap.
6. Store the individually wrapped bars in the fridge or freezer. They will be very chewy if stored in the fridge and have a little more snap to them if stored in the freezer. Yes, they can be eaten frozen.

Flour-less Sugarless Blueberry Muffins

Servings: 12 ❖ Calories per serving: 139

This recipe is gluten-free but does contain eggs and dairy. It makes lovely, moist muffins.

Ingredients:

- 1 cup firm whole milk yogurt
- 2 eggs
- ½ cup honey
- 1½ teaspoons baking powder
- ½ teaspoon baking soda
- 2½ cups rolled oats
- 1½ cups blueberries, fresh or frozen

Directions:

1. Pre-heat the oven to 400°F.
2. Spray muffin tins with non-stick cooking spray.

   Note: DO NOT use paper liners. They don't work well with flour-less recipes.

3. Combine the first six ingredients (everything except the blueberries) in a blender or food processor and blend until the mixture is smooth.

   Note: When using a blender, I have found that putting the liquid/moist ingredients in first works best. Then add the rolled oats, half a cup at a time, so not to overwork the blender.

4. Pour the mixture into a large bowl and stir in the blueberries.

   Note: the mixture will seem very liquid but will also been fairly sticky.

5. Spoon about ¼ cup of batter into each of the 12 muffin tins.
6. Bake at 400°F for 20-25 minutes, or until a toothpick inserted in the center comes out clean.

   Note: watch them carefully when they are getting close to done. Anything with honey in it burns easily.

7. Remove from the oven and cool on a wire rack. Allow the muffins to cool about 5-10 minutes before removing from muffin tins. Then allow the muffins to cool completely on a wire rack.

Sugar-Free, Gluten-Free, Egg-Free, Oil-Free Strawberry Muffins

Servings: 12 ❖ Calories per serving: 88

This recipe started as a way to eliminate sugar from a muffin recipe that we really liked and then evolved to cover a lot of scenarios that friends and family had been asking about. So we developed the recipe to also eliminate gluten, eggs and oil. The muffins are still wonderful and are vegan and low calories to boot.

Ingredients:

- 1 tablespoon ground flax seed
- 4 tablespoons water
- ⅔ cup sorghum flour
- ⅔ cup chickpea flour
- 1 cup gluten free quick oats
- 1 tablespoon baking powder
- ½ teaspoon sea salt
- ½ teaspoon cinnamon
- 1 cup rice milk
- 3 tablespoons unsweetened apple sauce
- 1 teaspoon vanilla
- 1 cup strawberries, fresh or frozen, diced

Directions:

1. Pre-heat oven to 350°F and grease a muffin tin (makes 12).
2. In a small bowl, combine the ground flax seed and water. Stir well and set aside. (This makes an egg substitute.)
3. In a large mixing bowl, combine the sorghum flour, chickpea flour, oats, baking powder, salt and cinnamon. Mix well.
4. In a separate bowl or measuring cup, combine the rice milk, applesauce, vanilla and flax seed mixture. Stir well.
5. Stir the liquid mixture into the dry mixture and mix just enough so that the dry ingredients are well moistened. Then fold in the diced strawberries.
6. Divide the batter evenly between the 12 muffin cups.
7. Bake at 350°F for 30-35 minutes or until a toothpick inserted in the center comes out clean and muffins are slightly browned.
8. Remove the muffins from the oven and cool on a wire rack for about 10 minutes. Remove the muffins from the muffin tin and allow them to continue cooling on the wire rack.
9. Any leftover muffins will freeze well.

Potato Skins

Servings: 16 ❖ Calories per serving: 160

Potato skins are popular in pubs, but you can make them at home, too. You can either leave the skins whole or, after they are completed, slice them in halves or thirds to make them more appetizer size. The bacon in this recipe is optional.

Ingredients:

    4 large Russet potatoes, baked
    3 tablespoons olive oil
    1 tablespoon parmesan cheese, grated
    ½ teaspoon sea salt, freshly ground
    ¼ teaspoon garlic powder
    ⅛ teaspoon black pepper, freshly ground
    8 strips bacon, cooked and crumbled (optional)
    2 cups cheddar cheese, shredded
    ½ cup sour cream
    4 green onions, sliced

Directions:

1. Pre-heat the oven to 450°F.
2. Cut already-baked and cooled potatoes in half lengthwise.
3. Scoop out most of the white pulp, leaving about ¼ inch of potato in the shell.
4. You can either discard the potato pulp or keep it for another use (like having it for dinner!).
5. Place the potato skin shells on a greased baking sheet.
6. In a small bowl, mix together the oil, Parmesan cheese, salt, garlic powder and pepper.
7. Using a pastry brush, brush the mixture over the potato skins, inside and out.
8. Bake at 450°F for about 8 minutes, then turn the skins over and bake for another 8 minutes.
9. Remove from oven and turn the skins right side up. Sprinkle each potato skin evenly with the crumbled bacon (if using) and the shredded cheddar cheese.
10. Return to oven and bake for another 2 minutes or until the cheese is melted.
11. Remove from oven and cool slightly on a wire rack.
12. Top with the sour cream and sliced green onions.

Raw Veggies and Dip

Servings: 4 ❖ Calories per serving: 171 (may vary slightly depending on type of hummus used)

This is a very simple recipe but one that, we've found, most people don't tend to do. This is a great idea for a snack or even an evening meal. Who says the vegetables have to be cooked just because it's suppertime?

Ingredients:

4 ribs celery
2 medium carrots
½ head cauliflower
1 head broccoli
4 spring onions
½ medium cucumber
½ medium red bell pepper
½ cup sugar snap peas
½ cup fresh green beans
1 cup hummus, for dip (three recipes for hummus follow)

Directions:

1. Clean all of the vegetables and cut into bite-size pieces.
2. We like to vary how we cut them up and do things like cut the carrots into matchsticks, the cauliflower and broccoli into flowerets, the cucumber into spears - you get the idea.
3. Provide each person with their own small dish of hummus to use as a dip.
4. That's it - easy and healthy!

Geoff's Famous Hummus
Servings: 24 ❖ Calories per serving: 21

Geoff is our hummus maker extraordinaire and he loves to experiment. This is his "famous" recipe. Very, very tasty.

Ingredients:
- 1 can chickpeas, 15 ounces, drained, reserve liquid
- 1 ounce sun dried tomatoes, NOT packed in water or oil
- ½ lime, juice only
- 3 cloves garlic
- 6 slices jalapeno, or to taste
- 3 teaspoons tahini paste
- ½ teaspoon sea salt
- ½ teaspoon freshly ground black pepper
- 1 tablespoon balsamic vinegar

Directions:
1. Place all ingredients, in order listed, in a food processor and blend until smooth.
2. Add reserved liquid as required to achieve desired consistency. You'll probably need about half of the liquid.

CREAMY DILL HUMMUS

Servings: 24 ❖ Calories per serving: 23

This is a light, creamy, fresh-tasting hummus. It works great as a dip and also as a spread for crackers or sandwiches. Makes for a killer tomato sandwich.

INGREDIENTS:

- 1 can chickpeas, 15 ounces, drained
- 3 tablespoons tahini paste
- 1 large kosher dill pickle, chopped
- 2 sprigs fresh dill

DIRECTIONS:

1. Combine all ingredients in a food processor and blend until smooth.

Spicy Jalapeno Dill Hummus
Servings: 24 ❖ Calories per serving: 27

In this recipe we've used chickpeas that we cooked from dried. If you use canned chickpeas, be sure to drain and rinse them. Also, with canned chickpeas, you may need less liquid.

Ingredients:
- 2 cups chickpeas
- 2 large kosher dill
- 2 tablespoons balsamic vinegar
- ¼ cup dill juice
- ¼ teaspoon salt
- 5 pickled jalapeno slices

Directions:
1. Place all of the ingredients in a food processor and blend until smooth.

Extras

This "Extras" section is for recipes that didn't neatly fit into the other categories of this book but that you might like to have as well.

Vegetable Broth

Believe it or not, most commercially produced vegetable broths have sugar in them - yes, sugar! So, here's how we can make our own vegetable broth.

> *Hint: Freeze some of the vegetable broth in ice cube trays and just use as needed, directly from the freezer.*

There's really no recipe for this. The best thing to do is to save all the water from boiling or steaming vegetables. In addition to that, try boiling down any peelings and bits that have been cut off vegetables before cooking, like broccoli bottoms and carrots tops and bottoms.

This kind of vegetable broth is just that - broth. No sugar, no spices, nothing but honest-to-goodness veggie nutrients in water.

Bread Machine Rye Bread

Servings: 24 (12 slices per loaf) ❖ Calories per serving: 115

This is one of our favorite rye bread recipes and we have made it both with and without the caraway seeds. It makes a great sandwich bread and toasts well, too.

In this recipe we use a 3 lb. bread machine to make the dough and then bake two one-and-a-half pound loaves in the oven.

Ingredients:

- 2¼ cups water, warm
- 2 teaspoons salt
- 3 tablespoons oil olive
- ¼ cup honey
- 2 cups unbleached all-purpose flour
- 2 cups whole wheat flour
- 1 cup rye flour
- 1 tablespoon yeast
- 1½ tablespoons caraway seed, optional

Directions:

1. Add all ingredients, with the exception of the caraway seeds, to the bread pan in the order suggested by the bread machine manufacturer.
2. Select the dough setting and press start.
3. Add the caraway seeds at the "add-in" beep.
4. Remove the dough from bread machine and knead for 2-3 minutes on a lightly floured surface.
5. Divide dough in half and place in two lightly greased loaf pans. Cover each loaf pan with plastic.
6. Allow the bread dough to rise, in a warm place, for about an hour.

Note: *an oven with just the interior light on is the perfect temperature for allowing bread dough to rise.*

7. After you have removed the risen loaves from the oven, turn the oven on and heat to 350°F.
8. Bake the loaves at 350°F for 30 to 35 minutes or until the loaves are well browned and sound hollow when tapped on the bottom.
9. Remove the loaves from the oven and remove the loaves from the loaf tins (they should come out easily). Then allow the loaves to cool completely on a wire rack. Bread slices best when it is cool.

Whole Wheat Sunflower Seed Bread
Servings: 24 (12 slices per loaf) ❖ Calories per serving: 130

The sunflower seeds give this bread a lovely nutty taste and the wheat bran adds additional fiber. This loaf freezes well and is good for both sandwiches and toasting.

In this recipe we use a 3 lb. bread machine to make the dough and then bake two one-and-a-half pound loaves in the oven.

Ingredients:
- 2 cups warm water
- 2 tablespoons dry buttermilk powder
- 3 tablespoons olive oil
- 4 tablespoons honey
- 2 teaspoons sea salt
- 3 cups whole wheat flour
- 1½ cups unbleached all-purpose flour
- 1 cup wheat or oat bran
- 2½ teaspoons active dry yeast
- ½ cup sunflower seeds

Directions:
1. Add all ingredients, with the exception of the sunflower seeds, to the bread pan in the order suggested by the bread machine manufacturer.
2. Select the dough setting and press start.
3. Add the sunflower seeds at the "add-in" beep.
4. Remove the dough from bread machine and knead for 2-3 minutes on a lightly floured surface.
5. Divide dough in half and place in two lightly greased loaf pans. Cover each loaf pan with plastic.
6. Allow the bread dough to rise, in a warm place, for about an hour.
7. After the loaves have risen, bake at 350°F for 30 to 35 minutes or until the loaves are well browned and sound hollow when tapped on the bottom.
8. Remove the loaves from the oven and remove the loaves from the loaf tins (they should come out easily). Then allow the loaves to cool completely on a wire rack. Bread slices best when it is cool.

Easy Buttermilk Biscuits

Servings: 12 ❖ Calories per serving: 124

Biscuits are always a nice addition to just about any meal - breakfast, lunch or dinner. These ones are easy to make and turn out great.

Ingredients:
- 2 cups unbleached all-purpose flour
- ¼ cup extra virgin olive oil
- 3 teaspoons baking powder
- 1 teaspoon baking soda
- 1 cup buttermilk or sour milk

Directions:
1. Pre-heat the oven to 400°F. Lightly grease a baking sheet and set aside.
2. In a large bowl, combine the flour, olive oil, baking powder, baking soda and milk.
3. Stir with a wooden spoon until the mixture forms a smooth batter.
4. Drop by rounded tablespoons onto the prepared baking sheet.
5. Bake at 400°F for 10 to 15 minutes, until golden brown.

STIR FRY SAUCE #1

Servings: 4 ❖ Calories per serving: 77

This stir fry sauce is quick and easy and done in the microwave. A great sauce for anything you care to stir fry.

INGREDIENTS:
- ¼ cup soy sauce
- 1 tablespoon balsamic vinegar
- ¼ cup honey
- ½ cup vegetable broth
- ¼ teaspoon cayenne pepper

DIRECTIONS:
1. Place all ingredients in a microwave-safe measuring cup and microwave on high for 20 seconds or until honey is well incorporated into the sauce. Stir well.

Stir Fry Sauce #2

Servings: 4 ❖ Calories per serving: 73
(with dates), 40 (without dates)

Some of us like our stir fry sauce a little sweeter than others. In this recipe the dates, as well as the red pepper flakes are optional. The dates, however, more than double the calorie count of this sauce. In addition to that there is, naturally, fructose in the dates and because the sauce is being blended smooth, a lot of the effect of the fiber in the dates is diminished. But don't panic, all the fiber in the vegetables that go into the stir fry will offset any negative effect from the fructose.

Ingredients

   2 cups vegetable broth
   ¼ cup soy sauce
   3 tablespoons cornstarch
   1 inch fresh ginger, piece, minced
   4 cloves garlic, minced
   2 Medjool dates, chopped, optional
   ¼ teaspoon red pepper flakes, optional

Directions:

1. Combine all ingredients in a food processor and blend until smooth.

Warm Horseradish Sauce

Servings: 2 ❖ Calories per servings: 44

We love making a vegetarian "meat" loaf. We also like to have a sauce to go with it. One of our favorite things when we were meat-eaters was horseradish. We hated to give up this lovely condiment and have found many uses for it in our vegetarian diet. Here's a warm, sugar-free, dairy-free version of a horseradish sauce. Be sure to use a good horseradish.

Ingredients:

½ cup almond milk
2½ tablespoons horseradish, grated
¼ teaspoon Dry mustard
1 ½ teaspoons garlic, minced
1 tablespoon cornstarch
1 tablespoon almond milk

Directions:

1. In a small saucepan, combine the almond milk, horseradish, dry mustard and garlic. Stir, with a wooden spoon or whisk, to combine.
2. Cook over medium heat just to a simmer.
3. Combine the tablespoon of corn starch with the ½ tablespoon of almond milk and mix well until smooth.
4. Slowly drizzle the corn starch mixture into the saucepan and stir constantly until the sauce becomes smooth and thickened.
5. Remove from heat and serve immediately.

Roasted Garlic Salad Dressing
Servings: 12 ❖ Calories per serving: 87

Making our own salad dressings is not only easy, but it ensures that we get the freshest dressing without any added sugar or preservatives. And, it just plain tastes better!

Note: *Instructions on how to roast the garlic follow.*

INGREDIENTS:
- 2 heads roasted garlic, peeled
- ½ cup extra virgin olive oil
- ¼ cup apple cider vinegar, with "The Mother"
- 2 tablespoons lemon juice, freshly squeezed
- ½ teaspoon kosher salt
- 1 teaspoon black pepper
- 1 tablespoon honey

DIRECTIONS:
1. Add all the ingredients to a food processor or blender and process until smooth.
2. Refrigerate until ready to serve and shake well before serving.

Hint: This dressing also makes a good marinade for grilled or roasted vegetables and even chicken or pork, if you eat meat.

How to Roast Garlic

DIRECTIONS:
1. Use complete heads of garlic.
2. With a sharp knife, carefully slice off the top of the garlic, just enough to expose the very top of each clove.
3. Drizzle each head with about 1 teaspoon of olive oil, trying to make sure that each of the cloves gets some of the oil.
4. For roasting just a couple of heads, place each head in a ceramic ramekin and cover with foil.
5. For roasting several heads at one time, use a muffin tin and cover each head with foil.
6. For roasting a small number of heads, pre-heat a toaster oven to 400°F and roast the garlic heads for 30 - 45 minutes until they are soft and slightly browned.
7. For roasting a large number of head, pre-heat a regular oven to 400°F and roast the garlic heads, in a muffin tin, for 30-45 minutes until they are soft and slightly browned.
8. Allow them to cool. Once cool the roasted cloves should come out easily either by squeezing each clove or by peeling them.

Hint: When we make garlic toast, we like to spread mashed, roasted garlic on the toast - no butter. It tastes great!

Adjust Your Own Recipes

You may find it surprisingly easy to adjust some of your own recipes to eliminate sugar and/or packaged ingredients. Often, honey or maple syrup are good substitutions, but a paste of boiled dates or boiled prunes is very sweet too, as is unsweetened applesauce.

We encourage you to experiment. Will every recipe work out? No. But there may be an award winning recipe just waiting to be discovered thanks to your willingness to "think outside the box."

Free Gift Now
+ Get Free Books Later

As a special thank you for purchasing this book we want to give you a free gift. Just visit this secret web page and pick up your free copy of "Our Favorite Detox and Weight Loss Slow Cooker Recipes"

http://ebooks.geezerguides.com/your-free-gift/

Also, each time any of our current or new books are offered for free, we'll be sure to tell you and hope you would take the time to review some of them.

One of the toughest things for an independent author is to get honest reviews for their books. We will gladly notify you of the availability of free copies of our books in hopes that, if you like them, you will post an honest review.

There's no catch and no obligation, just check the box on our website. Thank you. (We promise - NO SPAM - we hate it too)

Please Review Break Your Sugar Addiction Recipes

Now that you've reached the end of the this book, we would really appreciate you taking a moment to post a review on your local Amazon site: Just use the URL below to reach this book's page on Amazon.

http://geni.us/TNR2

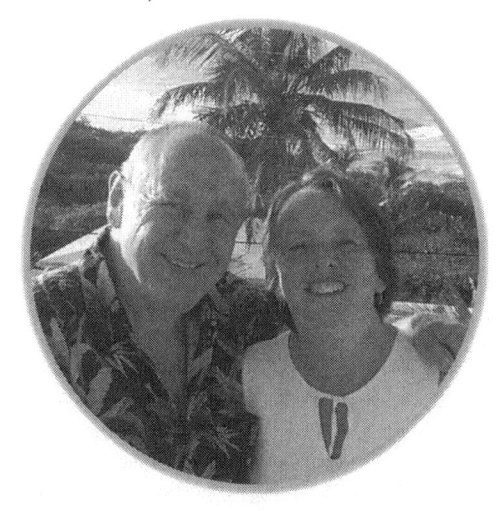

About The Authors

Geoff and Vicky Wells are real people who have real lives. They are a retired computer programmer (Geoff) and customer service consultant (Vicky). They spend summers in Northern Canada and winters in the Bahamas.

They write books on many subjects under various pen names. Mostly healthy living and cookbooks but also children's books, science fiction and anti-establishment rants.

If you want to know more please visit http://geoffandvickywells.com

The site is often out of date, incomplete and not particularly interesting but you are welcome to check it out. Much the same can be said for the blog at http://geezerguides.com

The most interesting site is at http://terranovian.com but if you visit be warned that you may be turned into a raving activist and get banned from all your friends cocktail parties.

We also have author pages on Amazon

http://amazon.com/author/vickyjwells

http://amazon.com/author/geoffwells

Contact Us

Life keeps us quite busy but we try to keep up with posts on several social networks and we welcome you to join us. If you visit please "Like" the page.

Facebook

https://www.facebook.com/pages/The-Terra-Novian-Way/179965592154046

https://www.facebook.com/GeezerGuides

https://www.facebook.com/ReluctantVegetarians

Twitter

http://twitter.com/TerraNovianWay

http://twitter.com/GeezerGuides

https://twitter.com/NutritiousFood

Goodreads

https://www.goodreads.com/author/show/5442787.Geoff_Wells

https://www.goodreads.com/author/show/2864210.Vicky_Wells

Shelfari

http://www.shelfari.com/authors/a1002691403/Geoff-Wells/

Google+

https://plus.google.com/104962434482327095816/posts

YouTube

https://www.youtube.com/channel/UCw-aid2E0NB8nUcLjUfiYeA

MORE BOOKS FROM GEEZER GUIDE PUBLISHING

The companion book to this one is "Sugar and the Evil Empire". If you want to know all about sugar, its history, who profits from it, how it effects your body and how you can avoid it - this is a book you need to read.

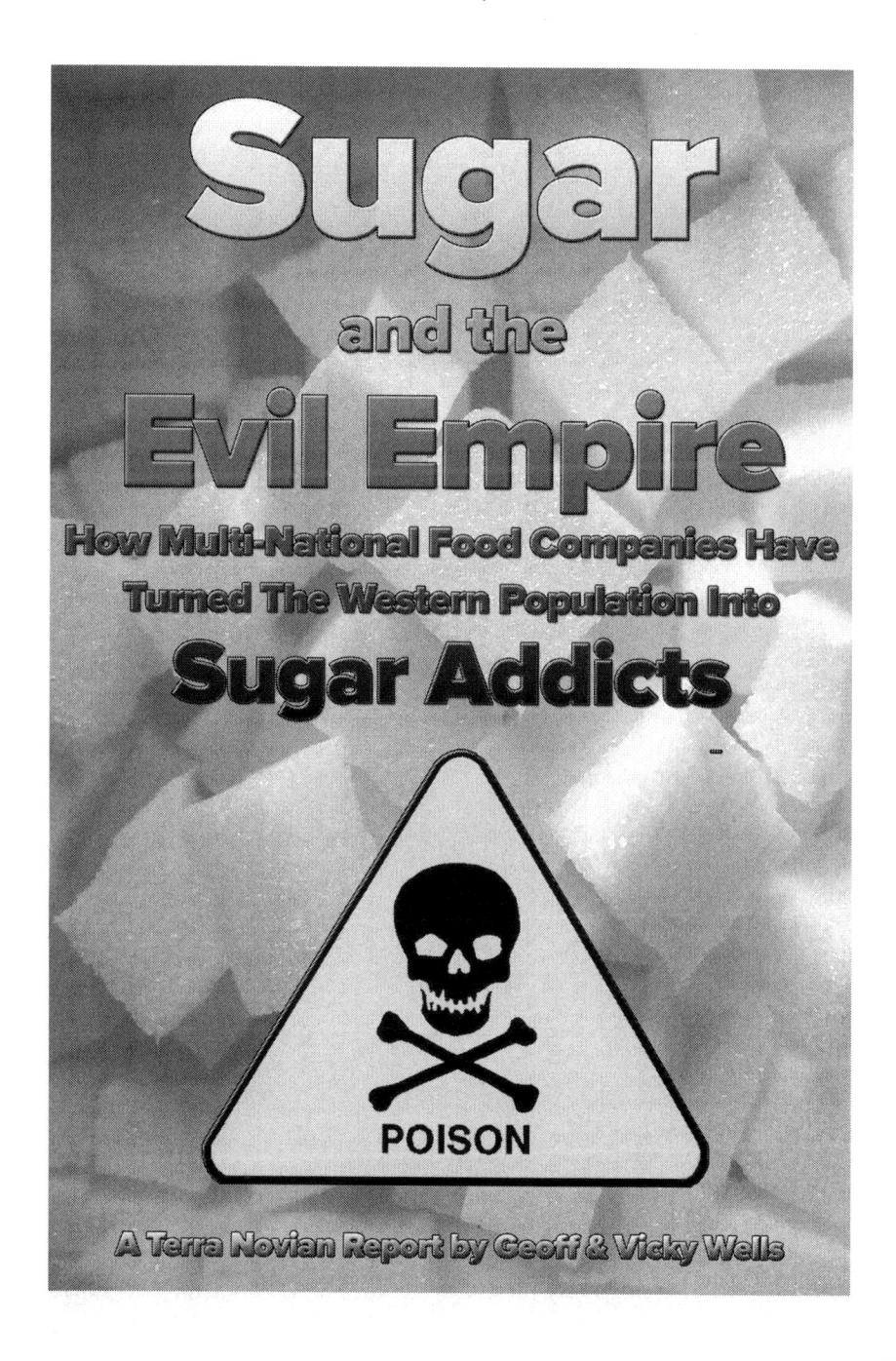

Sugar and the Evil Empire
How Multi-National Food Companies Have Turned The Western Population Into Sugar Addicts

A Terra Novian Report by Geoff & Vicky Wells

Printed in Great Britain
by Amazon